DEMOCRATISATION IN THE AGE OF AIDS

Understanding the political implications

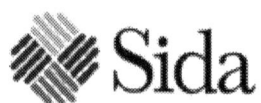

Sida   *id*asa

This publication has been produced with the support of SIDA. The content of the publication is the sole responsibility of IDASA and can in no way be taken to reflect the views of SIDA.

First published 2006

ISBN 1-920118-23-3   ISBN-13: 978-1-920118-23-5

Published by the Institute for Democracy in South Africa (IDASA)
6 Spin St, Cape Town, South Africa, 8001
Cnr Prinsloo and Visagie Streets, P.O Box 56950, Arcadia 0007
Pretoria, South Africa

www.idasa.org.za

Production by IDASA Publishing

Cover by Magenta Media

Printed by Lightning Source

DEMOCRATISATION IN THE AGE OF AIDS

Understanding the political implications

Kondwani Chirambo

2006

The Governance and AIDS Programme Staff

Kondwani Chirambo, Programme Manager

Marietjie Myburg, Regional Media Coordinator

Josina Machel, Capacity-Building Coordinator

Rabelani Daswa, Trainer and Researcher, AIDS Budget Unit (ABU)

Christele Dewouta, Intern

Vasanthie Naicker, Administrator

Acknowledgments

The Governance and AIDS Programme (GAP) wishes to thank the Swedish International Development Agency (SIDA) for the generous support that has enabled us to conduct this multi-country study. The SIDA grant builds on the funding provided by the Rockefeller Brothers Fund and the Ford Foundation before it, in developing what has become an important policy tool in dealing with the HIV/AIDS pandemic.

This work, which has been shared with important political actors in Africa and abroad, has provided a strong basis to renew efforts at strengthening the role of political institutions in the management of the pandemic and in governance more generally. Through national and regional dialogue forums, the consequences of AIDS for governance are being increasingly understood as the empirical data emerges.

We see a great potential in developing important follow-ups to address many facets around the leadership of the pandemic and the strategic visions required to address the dire situation of the current and future generations.

The multi-country studies afford us an opportunity to understand for the first time the impact of HIV/AIDS on elected leaders, political institutions and on citizen participation in ways which fundamentally challenge traditional approaches to combating HIV/AIDS and its side effects of stigma and discrimination.

Our aim is to collectively build strategies with African leaders as part of our contribution to the noble cause of defeating the pandemic. In this regard, we thank the many representatives of governments, parliaments, political parties, People Living with HIV/AIDS (PLWHAS), electoral commissions, regional bodies and inter-governmental agencies that have participated in the pre- and post-research stakeholder meetings held in Botswana, Namibia, Malawi, Tanzania, South Africa, Senegal and Zambia.

The multi-country studies are being undertaken with local partners. In this report some of the preliminary findings of the IDASA multi-country studies undertaken with the Center for Social Research (CSR) at the University of Malawi; the Namibia Institute for Democracy (NID); the Economic and Social Research Foundations in Tanzania (ESRF); and the Foundation for Democratic Processes (FODEP) in Zambia are shared along with findings from our pilot and South Africa studies. Other institutions involved in the study are the Southern African Centre for Policy Dialogue and Development (SACPODD) and the Institute for Environmental Sciences at the University of Cheik Anta Diop, Dakar, Senegal.

With the support of all stakeholders, we the staff of IDASA-GAP believe we can, together, make a major difference in building new knowledge and strategies on how to curtail the devastating course of the HIV/AIDS pandemic.

Kondwani Chirambo
Manager
Governance and AIDS Programme

HIV/AIDS prevalence in sub-Saharan Africa, 2005

Source: UNAIDS 2006 Global Report

About the author

Kondwani Chirambo is the Manager of the Governance and AIDS Programme (GAP) of the Institute for Democracy in South Africa (IDASA). GAP researches the impact of HIV/AIDS on democracy in several African countries. Chirambo initiated the AIDS and Elections Project for IDASA in 2003 and wrote the first research paper to provide empirical evidence on the impact of HIV/AIDS on the electoral process, focusing on Zambia, in 2003. He developed this pilot project into a multi-country study covering Botswana, Namibia, Malawi, South Africa, Tanzania, Senegal and Zambia. The AIDS and Elections Project now involves several distinguished academics and research institutions in Africa and is engaged in national and regional policy initiatives aimed at developing new political approaches to dealing with HIV/AIDS. Chirambo holds a Master of Arts Degree in Mass Communications from the University of Leicester, United Kingdom; an Advanced Diploma in Human Rights Law from the Raoul Wallenberg Institute, University of Lund, Sweden; and a three-year Diploma in Journalism from the Evelyn Hone College of Applied Arts and Commerce, Lusaka, Zambia. Chirambo is a doctoral candidate in Communication Science with the University of South Africa (UNISA).

Tel: 27-12-3920500/556
Cell: 072-1711808
E-mail: kchirambo@idasa.org.za
P.O. Box 56950
Cnr Prinsloo and Visagie Streets
Arcadia 0007
Pretoria
South Africa

Abbreviations

ACDP	African Christian Democratic Party (South Africa)
AFD	Alliance for Democracy (Malawi)
ANC	African National Congress (South Africa)
ART	Antiretroviral treatment
ARVs	Antiretrovirals
CSR	Center for Social Research (Malawi)
DA	Democratic Alliance (DA)
EMB	Electoral Management Body
ESRF	Economic and Social Research Foundation (Tanzania)
EU	European Union
FODEP	Foundation for Democratic Processes (Zambia)
FPTP	First-Past-the-Post (electoral system)
GAP	Governance and AIDS Programme (South Africa)
GNP	Gross National Product
HSRC	Human Sciences Research Council (South Africa)
IDASA	Institute for Democracy in South Africa
IEC	Independent Electoral Commission (South Africa)
IFP	Inkatha Freedom Party (South Africa)
INERSOR	Institute for Economic and Social Research (Zambia)
MCP	Malawi Congress Party
MEC	Malawi Electoral Commission
MIM	Malawi Institute of Management
MMD	Movement for Multi-party Democracy (Zambia)
MMP	Mixed-Member Proportional (electoral system)
MP	Member of Parliament
NEPAD	New Partnership for Africa's Development
NIS	Namibia Institute for Democracy

PLWHAs	People Living With HIV/AIDS
PR	Proportional Representation (electoral system)
RBF	Rockefeller Brothers Fund
SACPDODD	Southern African Centre for Policy Dialogue and Development
SADC	Southern African Development Community
SADC-ECF	SADC Electoral Commissions Forum
SARDC	Southern African Research and Documentation Centre
SIDA	Swedish International Development Cooperation Agency
SMM	Single-Member Majority (electoral system)
SMP	Single-Member Plurality (electoral system)
TAPAC	Tanzania Parliamentarians AIDS Coalition
TAC	Treatment Action Campaign (South Africa)
UDF	United Democratic Front (Malawi)
UNAIDS	Joint United Nations Programme on HIV/AIDS
UNDP	United Nations Development Programme
UNIP	United National Independence Party (Zambia)
UNECA	United Nations Economic Commission for Africa
VCT	Voluntary Counselling and Testing
ZESN	Zimbabwe Election Support Network

Contents   Page

Tables   Page

Figures
Page

Introduction

Project profile

The Institute for Democracy in South Africa's (IDASA's) Governance and AIDS Programme (GAP) holds the distinction of being the first research unit anywhere to establish the empirical link between HIV/AIDS and democratic governance, using the electoral process as an entry point. Based on its ground-breaking research, GAP has begun a process of developing strategic approaches for political leaders/policy-makers as a contribution to the effective management of the pandemic. This project, funded by the Swedish International Development Cooperation Agency (SIDA), is being conducted simultaneously in six African countries: Namibia, Malawi, Zambia, Tanzania, Botswana and Senegal. It is a follow-up to the pilot study in Zambia in 2003 funded by the Ford Foundation and subsequent research in South Africa undertaken in 2004/5 supported by the Rockefeller Brothers Fund (RBF).

The AIDS and Elections Project – one of four projects of IDASA-GAP – is an initiative that emerged from consultations with political agencies at the highest level. The Electoral Commissions Forum of SADC Countries (SADC-ECF) in particular emphasised the importance of such research to mitigate post-election conflict. This emerged at IDASA-GAP's April 2003 Governance and AIDS Forum which was supported by SIDA, the European Union (EU) and the United Nations Development Programme (UNDP) (Ngwembe, in Chirambo and Caesar. 2003). The SADC-ECF is the association of all Electoral Management Bodies (EMBs) in Southern Africa. The Governance and AIDS Forum also involved senior representatives from UNDP and Joint United Nations Programme on HIV/AIDS (UNAIDS) country offices, the SADC Parliamentary Forum, the SADC Health Sector Coordinating Unit, civil society and donor agencies. The presidency of South Africa officiated at the Forum.

The available evidence suggests that the threat of AIDS remains real, devastating and all-pervading. It encompasses all spheres of life. It spares nothing; not even politics.

This publication presents the results of three principal research projects, all of them complimentary and ground-breaking.

* The findings of the pilot project in Zambia (2003);
* The key findings of the South African study (2005);
* The preliminary findings of the multi-country study of six African countries (2006).

The purpose of the study is to establish the impact of HIV/AIDS on the electoral process using democratic governance as the analytical concept. The outcomes are shared with relevant state and non-state actors for capacity building and policy interventions. The political institutions which form the focus of this research all play a critical role in the quality of governance and contribute to political stability and legitimacy. We focus on electoral systems because they determine power configurations in decision-making processes, influencing the level of diversity and therefore inclusivity in the setting of national priorities, including policy priorities on AIDS matters (Reynolds, et al, 2005).[i] Political parties articulate the varied interests of society, foster representation and mobilise public support for governance priorities, and in many ways bring democratic accountability to bear on government, including on matters of health. Parliaments represent the political will and interests of the electorate; they deliberate on national priorities as representatives of the people – passing legislation and overseeing government action in many governance areas. They are, in addition, indispensable to the notion of "popular self government" on which democracies ride. Electoral commissions lie at the heart of a stable democracy, lending credibility and integrity to the democratic process by ensuring that the rules are applied fairly and that, to the extent possible, the majority of citizens participate freely in making policy choices, including AIDS policy. Adding the voices of the marginalised in policy forums is also a fundamental component of human development.

Without the support and participation of citizens, the legitimacy of political systems is in doubt. Our emphasis on citizen participation in governance processes in this regard was to determine to what extent, if at all, AIDS-related sickness and care-giving prevents people from adding their voices to the policy arena. These are the same citizens who would ordinarily respond to policy interventions for strengthening economic and social profiles of nation-states.

More than 40 of the 53 states in Africa have embraced democracy. We argue that democracies are sensitive systems of governance that place a high premium on service delivery. Our aim therefore is to help African governments embrace additional strategies that can assist the nascent democracies to absorb, and respond more effectively to, the political, economic and social shocks introduced by the pandemic, using, among other tools, this new knowledge.

Results

This multi-country research demonstrates that HIV/AIDS is not just a health crisis, but a pandemic that has implications for political legitimacy and stability. The research uses both qualitative and quantitative methods and the following results have emerged:

- The epidemic impacts adversely on plural majority electoral systems in Africa, particularly the Single-Member Plurality (SMP), generating increasing economic costs for resource-stressed nations;

- The study provides indicative evidence of attrition amongst elected leadership which has strong correlations to HIV/AIDS mortality within the general population;

- The findings suggest that AIDS generates a stigma that prevents disclosure among political leaders and may compromise concerted efforts against the disease by the elite;

- AIDS contributes to power and gender imbalances in decision-making process;

- Stigma and discrimination may prevent rural-based South African People Living With HIV and AIDS (PLWHAs) from participating in public voting. Focus group discussions with PLWHAs were held in KwaZulu-Natal, one of the high prevalence provinces in South Africa and should not be generalised to other regions or countries where communities are less discriminatory;

- Interviews with senior electoral officers confirm that high attrition because of AIDS among teachers who constitute the bulk of the support staff to EMBs might compromise the effectiveness with which elections are run;

- AIDS has reduced the pool of voters in South Africa and is complicating the management of voters' rolls in other African countries with less sophisticated technologies for deleting dead voters from the voter registers. This exacerbates perceptions of "ghost voting" and therefore precipitates post-election conflict.

Implications

The analysis and results show that HIV/AIDS may compromise the democratic project in Africa by increasing expenditure on the sustenance of the dominant SMP electoral models; possibly decreasing participation in public policy processes by citizens living with the virus; potentially harming the capacity of EMBs to conduct elections effectively; and posing new challenges for multi-party democracy. While most of these areas need further research, there is a general indication that the impact of the pandemic on politics and its institutions is severe, albeit silent. Policy recommendations are made in this regard. In addition to the South African study, anecdotes from the ongoing research in Botswana, Malawi, Namibia, Senegal, Tanzania and Zambia are also highlighted.

Problem and background

Democracy and the AIDS conundrum

Without doubt, AIDS remains one of the biggest challenges facing emerging democracies in Africa today. Governments continue to grapple with mounting deaths in adult populations in whom many of the skills required for development reside. Several sub-Saharan countries are now caught in what Barnett and Whiteside (2002) term the "second" and "third" waves of the pandemic – when opportunistic infections, illness and death manifest with abandon.[ii]

But while the challenge posed by AIDS to socioeconomic development has been widely researched and acknowledged, the threat to politics has been less understood for some time, giving rise to a plethora of conjectures that have predicted doomsday scenarios for democracy in Africa. Democracy has been described as a system "sensitive to performance," one likely to be jeopardised by poor economic indicators of the sort that HIV/AIDS generates through absenteeisms and deaths among the productive class (Youde, 2001).

Measured against the liberal democratic standards of the United States, African states have been categorised by many US scholars as either "pseudo-democracies", "virtual democracies", "illiberal democracies" or "electoral democracies" depending on their level of development, generally connoting a degree of weakness that renders them extremely vulnerable to internal and external factors (Mattes, 2003).[iii] When conflated with AIDS, these assumptions have been framed in apocalyptic terms by Western scholars, many of whom have tended to readily embrace stereotypes about the "fragility" of African states and their vulnerability to destabilising elements without a critical appreciation of the continent's political trajectory and its survivability against many odds over time.

Similar theoretical speculation by Western-dominated South African researchers has posited a scenario of complete and utter chaos: AIDS orphans resorting to crime (Schonteich, 2003a);[iv] increasing state responsibilities for a vice already out of control in some countries; wholesale dissatisfaction with incapacitated state institutions leading to loss of confidence in elected government; withdrawal from politics by the AIDS sick and loss of enthusiasm for political life by people living with the virus; and a general weakening of social cohesion.[v] Extreme views have even suggested that small states with high HIV prevalence, such as Botswana, could be wiped off the face of the earth! Invariably, state collapse has been envisaged.

One of the fundamental flaws in this approach is the failure to involve other African scholars in the problem definition to a great extent, leaving the emerging field of "AIDS and governance" research to be largely fuelled by Western prejudices about the future of democracy on this continent. After almost half a decade of scepticism, these worst-case scenarios are being re-framed as neither socio-economic studies nor socio-political research on the impact of AIDS provide empirical evidence of collapse or democratic reversal.

Regardless, the available evidence suggests that the threat of AIDS remains real, devastating and all-pervading. It encompasses all spheres of life. It spares nothing; not even politics.

These fears were crystallised a little more than a decade ago when the realisation that HIV/AIDS would pose some serious ramifications for the developmental agenda of the United Nations (UN) led to sensitisation programmes that geneated a growing consensus that the disease was more than just a health crisis. Its profound effects on the social-economic fabric of society elevated the disease to the status of a crisis affecting governance more broadly, a point that many now concede.

Figure 1: 25 Years of AIDS

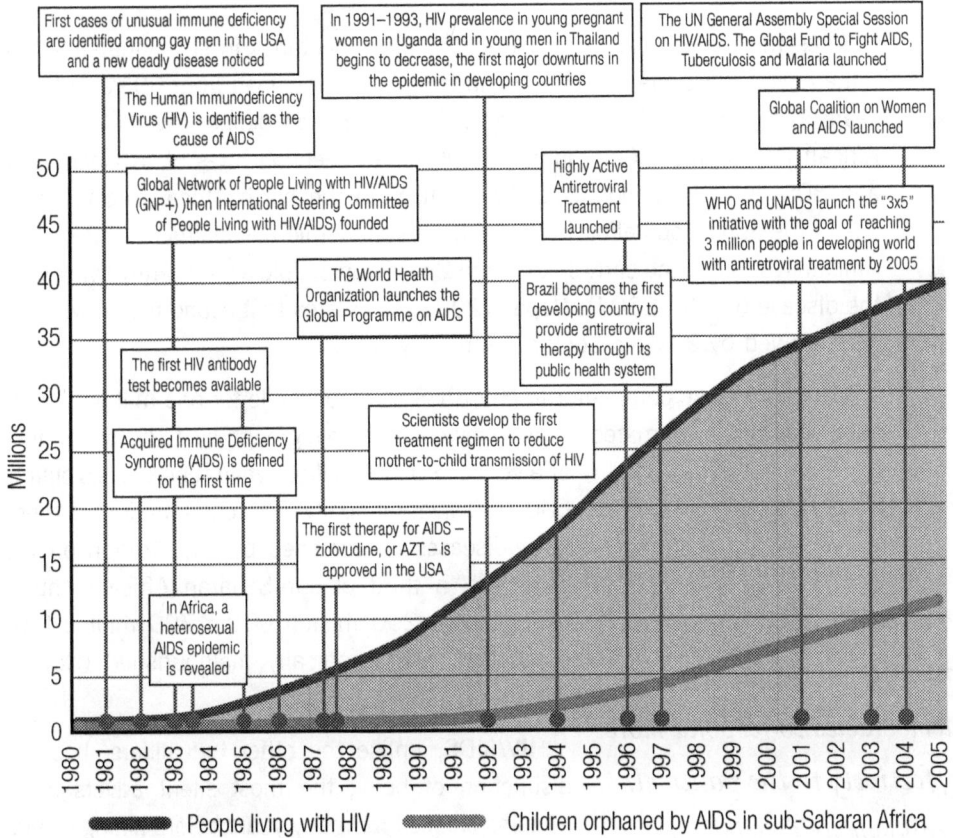

First cases of unusual immune deficiency are identified among gay men in the USA and a new deadly disease noticed

The Human Immunodeficiency Virus (HIV) is identified as the cause of AIDS

Global Network of People Living with HIV/AIDS (GNP+))then International Steering Committee of People Living with HIV/AIDS) founded

The World Health Organization launches the Global Programme on AIDS

The first HIV antibody test becomes available

Acquired Immune Deficiency Syndrome (AIDS) is defined for the first time

The first therapy for AIDS – zidovudine, or AZT – is approved in the USA

In Africa, a heterosexual AIDS epidemic is revealed

In 1991–1993, HIV prevalence in young pregnant women in Uganda and in young men in Thailand begins to decrease, the first major downturns in the epidemic in developing countries

Scientists develop the first treatment regimen to reduce mother-to-child transmission of HIV

Brazil becomes the first developing country to provide antiretroviral therapy through its public health system

Highly Active Antiretroviral Treatment launched

The UN General Assembly Special Session on HIV/AIDS. The Global Fund to Fight AIDS, Tuberculosis and Malaria launched

Global Coalition on Women and AIDS launched

WHO and UNAIDS launch the "3x5" initiative with the goal of reaching 3 million people in developing world with antiretroviral treatment by 2005

People living with HIV — Children orphaned by AIDS in sub-Saharan Africa

Source: UNAIDS, 2006 Report on the Global AIDS epidemic

Figure 2: Mortality in SADC, 1970-2010

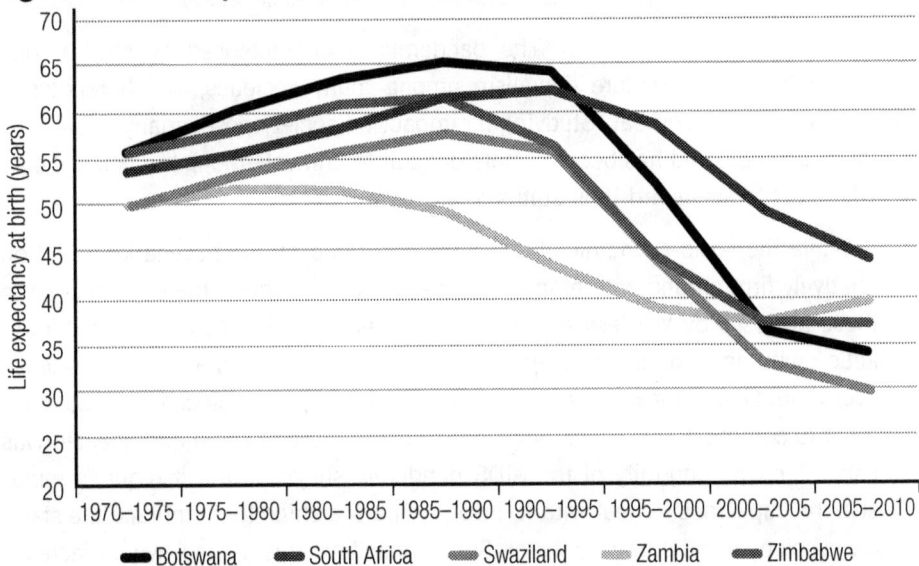

Botswana — South Africa — Swaziland — Zambia — Zimbabwe

Source: UNAIDS, 2006 Report on the Global AIDS epidemic

Since the materialisation of HIV/AIDS, life expectancy in sub-Saharan Africa – the region most affected by the pandemic – has declined from 60 years to 43 years in the most affected countries. The sub-region defined by the Southern African Development Community (SADC)[vi] has infection rates of between 15% and 30% in adult populations. In contrast, in the north African region about 1% of the adult population is infected. The pandemic has claimed 19.2 million African lives since the early 1980s and 25 million people are currently living with the disease (CHGA, 2004). Nepad (2003) calculates that economic growth has been slowed by 2.6% in Southern Africa by AIDS.

Malaria, a close competitor to HIV/AIDS, is responsible for one million deaths each year and is estimated to have slowed economic growth by 1.3% per annum at a cost of $US12 million while tuberculosis claims 600 000 lives annually. The combination of these killer diseases is worsened by malnutrition on the continent: a third of sub-Saharan Africans, numbering about 200 million of the 700 million total population, are chronically malnourished (Nepad, 2005).

Our aim is to help African governments embrace strategies that can assist the nascent democracies to respond more effectively to the political, economic and social shocks introduced by the pandemic.

HIV/AIDS, unlike the other two killers, has the distinction of being the most silent adversary. It remains cloaked for many years before killing its victims. It is mainly transmitted through sexual intercourse, which explains the taboos that accompany its prevalence in many societies.

The pandemic is characterised by stigma, discrimination and therefore denialism among many societies, which renders it more difficult to combat. Studying its impact on society poses many challenges for researchers and has become more difficult to unravel among the political elite who elect to safeguard their status at all costs.

While the socio-economic studies that illustrated the first scenarios stood on relatively firm ground with empirical evidence to back them, the political spin to these analyses by Western social scientists were based largely on limited interaction with and experience of African society, its institutions and their resilience over time. One thing was clear, however, AIDS required unprecedented commitment to combat it and a high degree of respect for the infected and affected was called for. The enormity of the AIDS pandemic suggests that it requires multi-sectoral capacities to deal with it, involving partnerships that embrace the state, civil society and the private sector. Such capacities, it is argued, would increase the potential for implementation, monitoring and evaluation of all interventions.

State, civil society and private sector partnerships

The application of the concept and process of governance to the management of the AIDS pandemic suggests that the disease is an immense development problem that cannot be handled by the state alone. In much of the literature, governance as a concept asserts a strategic developmental interaction between state and non-state actors in the management of political, economic and social affairs of a country.[vii] Based on this cross-sectoral collaboration, good governance is meant to deliver on many developmental fronts, including education and employment, allowing citizens to experience, among other things, long healthy lives and enabling them to express their policy choices.

HIV/AIDS is not just a health crisis, but a pandemic with implications for political legitimacy and stability.

More recently, UNDP has attached a normative edge to this concept by applying democratic values more critically. Good governance is now equated with democratic governance, embracing such institutions as freedom of expression and association, vibrant civil societies, gender equity and equality, the rule of law, fundamental human rights, media freedom, and free and fair elections. These elements, among several others, would be essential for the accountability and participation that are relevant to the practice of democracy and to the notion of effective governance of the pandemic. The re-evaluation of governance as a concept by UNDP has also more categorically endorsed democracy as the ideal system to provide the relevant environment for constructing responses that place citizens at the centre of all activity and nurture a viable alliance between state and non-state actors.[viii]

In other words, this would mean, among other things, that:

- People's human rights and fundamental freedoms are respected, allowing them to live in dignity (with a balance being between individual and group rights);

- There are inclusive and fair rules, institutions and practices that govern social interactions (including interaction between the infected and affected);

- People are free from discrimination based on race, ethnicity, class, gender and any other attribute (including HIV/AIDS status);

- The needs of a future generation are reflected in current practices (care for orphans and sustainability of society beyond the current generation);

- People can hold decision-makers accountable (several institutional arrangements may be used, democratic elections being one form);

- People have a say in decisions that affect their lives (they express their choice of policy for e.g. on HIV/AIDS in procedural processes, such as elections, among others) (Strand, et al. 2005).

In the wake of these theoretical discussions, the link between AIDS and govern-ance – and politics – as an activity of governance may still have been contestable. However, in 2003 IDASA published the results of a ground-breaking pilot study from Zambia (Chirambo, 2003; 2004) in which the first evidence of the impact of HIV/AIDS on key political institutions – electoral systems and parliament – emerged. IDASA followed this up with a more comprehensive comparative study of South Africa, Lesotho, Zambia and Zimbabwe (Strand, Matlosa, Strode and Chirambo, 2005) addressing the impact of HIV/AIDS on electoral processes.

Through GAP, IDASA has since launched a six-country comparative study covering Botswana, Namibia, Malawi, Tanzania, Senegal and Zambia with the involvement of local partners in each country. These research processes have been widely embraced by government, parliaments, research communities, civil societies and PLWHAs, underlining the relevance of socio-political research on AIDS.

Investigating HIV/AIDS and the electoral process

In our multi-country studies, we use the electoral process and the notions of "participation and accountability" to operationalise the UNDP definition of demo-cratic governance to understand the empirical link with HIV/AIDS.

The electoral process refers to both the system of rules governing elections and the implementation of those rules. Elections involve four sets of actors; political parties, EMBs, voters and parliament as an outcome. Elections and the electoral system – which constitute the methodology for arranging power in decision-mak-ing mechanisms – play an important role in determining the level of account-ability and representation in governance (Matlosa, 2003).

Using democratic governance as the central analytical concept, this project is therefore studying the impact of HIV/AIDS on the following key areas of the electoral process:

- Electoral systems: Their divergent strengths and weaknesses in the face of the HIV/AIDS epidemic;

- Electoral management and administration: The vulnerability of the EMBs to the effects of HIV/AIDS in both their internal functioning and their external mandate to deliver free and fair elections;

- Parliamentary configuration: Trends in mortality rates among parliamentarians in the pre-AIDS and post-AIDS eras, power shifts arising from by-elections held to replace deceased leaders;

- Political parties: The potential impact on political leadership and organising capacities;

- Voter and civic participation: Focus group discussions on the impact of stigma and discrimination from the perspective of PLWHAs.

Methodology

The research involved five different key methodological approaches to collecting information:

- A comprehensive overview of available literature, including an analysis of the legal and constitutional framework, the status of the voters' rolls with regard to deceased voters, and key epidemiological and electoral literature;

- Structured in-depth interviews with key informants, including political party officials and parliamentarians;

- Focus group discussions with PLWHAs – to augment the qualitative analysis of citizens' perceptions and assess their ability to participate in elections and civil society;

- Statistical analysis of public opinion survey data from the Afrobarometer to determine the impact HIV/AIDS has on civic participation and to correlate public perceptions with government actions; epidemiological and electoral data to determine the link between voter mortality and AIDS-related attrition in the general population;

- Post-research stakeholder meetings with state officials, researchers, political parties, UN agencies and other relevant organisations to review and validate outcomes.

Unfortunately the study has limitations. For one thing, we cannot ascertain the actual causes of deaths due to confidentiality clauses. Further, this research, like most in the social sciences, relies on proxy indicators to draw inferences on the possible influence of HIV/AIDS. This is also a largely unexplored field that requires immense resources to investigate thoroughly. Much of the evidence at this stage will therefore only be indicative. Lastly, poor record-keeping by public institutions and political parties compromises our ability to trace relevant data for a comprehensive analysis.

Overview of research outcomes

Given the increasing body of empirical evidence emerging from Southern Africa we can add more authority to some of the initial arguments we put forward and dispense with others. Clearly, there is no evidence of state collapse (National Intelligence Council, 2005), but many Africans will still die due to weak health systems, loss of health staff to AIDS and migration to Europe, limited coverage of Antiretroviral Treatment (ART) and poor nutrition, among other things. There are, however, some quite severe impacts affecting key political institutions which need critical attention. The following are the main empirical outcomes and common themes from the preliminary reports that will be elucidated in the succeeding narrative:

Without doubt, AIDS remains one of the biggest challenges facing emerging democracies in Africa today. Governments continue to grapple with mounting deaths in adult populations in whom many of the skills required for development reside.

• The dominant electoral system, SMP, also known as the First-Past-the-Post (FPTP) system, is being rendered economically unsustainable as deaths due to "long" and "short" illnesses mount among relatively young elected leaders. The multiple by-elections held to replace deceased leaders carry varied political and economic costs. The costs are most noticeable in countries with mature epidemics and relatively larger legislative bodies and national populations – Malawi, Zambia, Tanzania and Zimbabwe stand out;

• Constituencies that have had successive vacancies are being denied a voice in the development arena. The loss of representatives often leaves the districts without representation for long periods. In Malawi, it has taken up to 12 months to stage a by-election. Limited finances in countries that partly rely on donor support for elections are a possible explanation for the gaps between by-elections. Members of Parliament (MPs) report spending their own money on the funerals of deceased members of their constituencies, who see them as providers in every sense. This introduces a personal cost to the elected representative;

- AIDS is used as a political football, receiving high-level attention during elections which becomes denialism between polls. In Namibia, Malawi, South Africa and Zambia – four countries that have provided research results – there is fear and/or silence when it comes to disclosure of HIV status among elected leaders. Even though a handful of politicians have declared their negative status, there is not a single elected representative on record who lives with HIV/AIDS. The results fly in the face of the relatively high level of deaths amongst elected representatives which will be illustrated in this publication;

The pandemic is characterised by stigma, discrimination and therefore denialism among many societies, which renders it more difficult to combat.

- AIDS is being used as a political weapon in the electoral arena. Candidates perceived to be ill have been de-campaigned and maligned. The effect is that political parties are reluctant to adopt candidates who are or appear to be HIV-positive. This could have the effect of undermining efforts to deal with stigma and discrimination and discouraging a robust approach to dealing with it. It also seriously questions the already elusive concept of political commitment and how it can be applied to leaders who are in denial;

- Registered voter populations, particularly in the 30-49 age range in South Africa, have been dying in unusually large numbers. The mortality profiles are consistent with the pattern of deaths associated with AIDS and have occurred mainly in provinces with high HIV prevalence. The effect could compromise political party support bases. Other countries, such as Zambia, show a decline in voter populations in some – but not all – high HIV prevalence provinces. However there are other explanations for some of these phenomena, including labour migration resulting from the collapse of the privatisation programme in Zambia in the 1990s;

- Illness has already manifested itself as a problem amongst PLWHAs. Contrary to earlier assumptions that PLWHAs are likely to withdraw from political life, there seems to be recognition of the importance of elections as a means of adding their voices and enabling a choice of policy. This might also be explained by the fact that most PLWHAs who were willing to disclose their status were drawn from organisations of people living with the virus, who would be sensitised. However, there are structural and attitudinal factors that potentially stand in the way of PLWHAs and care-givers from accessing the vote, which include time constraints, physical challenges, distances to polling stations and lack of seating facilities at election centres. Stigma and discrimination were found to be a problem for rural registered voters in South Africa sampled in KwaZulu-Natal.

The effect of this enforced withdrawal from civic participation requires further investigation. No such concerns have been found thus far in other countries being studied, possibly because they have a longer history of HIV/AIDS education and therefore relatively less stigma in their communities;

- Without citizen and voter registration systems that are technologically sound and directly compatible, SADC governments will struggle to purge dead voters from their voters' registers, exposing elections to conflict over perceptions of "fraud" or "ghost voting". AIDS results in an increase in the number of dead voters on the roll and renders the register unmanageable if the necessary capacity is lacking. Controversy over the size of Malawi's voter population arose from a non-existent civic register and a disputed voters' roll. The Malawi electoral authority indicated that the number of voters on the voters' roll was not a true reflection of what was on the ground;

- There are noticeably high death levels among teachers and policemen/women who are normally deployed as part-time support staff by EMBs during elections. Studies undertaken by other institutions on the public service in Malawi and South Africa support this point. The retention of skills and experience appears to be being undermined;

- The weaknesses of political parties in Africa have again been underlined. Most are simply "election machines" designed to function as elections draw near. Their fragility is accentuated by the possibility that the patrons who finance and lead them will die young, taking their organisations with them. Some examples of this are known.[ix]

Registered voter populations, particularly in the 30-49 age range in South Africa, have been dying in unusually large numbers.

This new knowledge has had a sobering effect. We now know that the pandemic has stealthily depleted leadership and weakened some political institutions over a 20-year period, rendering some electoral systems unsustainable. Stigma and discrimination are being felt in the electoral arena and in people's daily lives, enforcing silent exclusion from normal life processes.

More importantly, though, we also know that something can be done to remedy the situation. In the next few pages, this discussion will be contextualised and some of the findings examined in greater detail, beginning with the electoral system.

Electoral systems: the link to governance

Defining electoral systems

Electoral systems are defined as the mechanisms that translate votes cast into seats and power in parliament and other decision-making structures. They also influence political party organisation and party systems in a country. Research shows for instance that Proportional Representation (PR) systems maximise the potential for gender and ethnic diversity therefore minimising conflict and fostering inclusivity in policy processes (Reynolds, et al, 2005). PR systems will often generate policy-based political parties. This is because inevitably the competing organisations need to appeal to the various interest and ethnic groups within the population to garner enough votes to gain seats in parliament. However, the PR system tends to be weak on accountability mainly because citizens elect political parties that in turn appoint representatives on the people's behalf. The power to appoint hence resides in the political party.

In the SMP system, also known as FPTP, political parties tend to be personality-based, without clear policy and ideological direction, and it is the strongest candidates and political parties that in the end claim a presence at constituency and national levels. As explained in greater detail below, this system is strong on accountability as leaders are directly elected by the voters.

An electoral system hence determines who is elected, how they are elected and who decides on national matters, including governance priorities concerning HIV/AIDS.

Electoral systems will have key variables, such as the electoral formula used (i.e. whether the system is majoritarian or proportional, what mathematical formula is used to calculate the seat allocation) and the district magnitude (how many members of parliament that district elects). The four main types of electoral systems employed in Southern Africa and their essential features are as follows:

Single-Member Plurality (SMP)

Popularly referred to as FPTP, this system is considered the simplest. The country is divided into electoral zones or constituencies and one candidate is chosen to represent each zone. The candidate who receives one more vote than the other contestants is declared victor, even if one does not obtain more votes than all the others combined. One of the key elements of this system is the requirement for a by-election or supplementary election to fill vacancies if the elected representative dies, resigns or crosses the floor. There are eight SADC countries that operate the FPTP electoral system: Botswana, Malawi, Mauritius, Seychelles, Swaziland, Tanzania, Zambia and Zimbabwe. Most of these are former British colonies.

Single-Member Majority (SMM)

The SMM system is similar to the SMP system in that the country is divided into electoral constituencies. However, the fundamental characteristic is that candidates are required to garner an absolute majority of votes (50 + 1%) in the constituency to be declared winner. Sometimes, where candidates fail to achieve an absolute majority, a run-off is called. The SMM has been used for presidential elections in some countries in the SADC region.

Proportional Representation (PR)

There are various types of PR systems worldwide but the most common is the closed party list system. Under this, the entire country constitutes a single constituency. Political parties will contest this space and will be allocated seats according to the proportion of votes they garner nationally. The PR system therefore favours broader representation. The parties will use the closed lists submitted to the EMBs to assign MPs to seats in hierarchical order. There is no requirement for a by-election when a vacancy occurs; rather parties fill the seat with the next person on the party list. The SADC member states that use the PR system are Angola, Mozambique, Namibia and South Africa.

Mixed-Member Proportional (MMP)

It has to be underlined that while South Africa uses the PR system at national level, it employs the MMP system at local government level. A combination of the PR and FPTP systems, it facilitates the election of one stream of MPs through the FPTP method and the other through the PR system. Only one SADC country has adopted the MMP system, Lesotho (EISA, 2003).

The link to HIV/AIDS

Because records on the actual causes of deaths of elected representatives are often unavailable, there are a number of steps we have taken to explain the impact of the AIDS pandemic on electoral systems:

- Comparing and analysing trends in the deaths of elected leaders in the "pre-AIDS" period and the "AIDS era";

- Analysing the age cohorts of the deceased (do they fall within the sexually active age group of 20-60 years?);

- Aggregating the causes of by-elections in countries that employ the FPTP system

(was there an increase in the number of by-elections caused by illness in the "AIDS era" compared to the "pre-AIDS era"?)

There are noticeably high death levels among teachers and policemen/ women who are normally deployed as part-time support staff by EMBs during elections.

Although these steps do not conclusively attribute deaths to AIDS they do help us draw inferences on the pattern of deaths and its similarity to the trends in the general population that has fallen to the disease. High mortality among younger politicians provides a strong basis to link the deaths that have been attributed officially to "long" or "short illness" to the influence of the pandemic.

Following this we expand the discussion by addressing the political and economic consequences of the pandemic resulting from its effect on the electoral system. These costs are best exemplified by assessing the FPTP and MMP systems which employ by-elections to fill vacancies. It is less useful to use the PR system because vacancies are filled by appointment from the lists. In understanding the political and economic costs therefore:

- We look at the loss of representation by constituencies as they await a new by-election;

- We analyse the potential impact on voters in terms of the fatigue accumulated from too many by-elections;

- Finally we calculate the financial costs of holding by elections.

Key findings: Impact of HIV/AIDS on electoral systems

By-elections in Zambia

Our pilot study undertaken in 2003 in Zambia – which uses the FPTP electoral method – indicates that between 1964 and 1984 (the 20-year period before the advent of HIV/AIDS) a total of 46 by-elections were held, 14 of them a result of death by illness and accidents combined. Over an 18-year period (from 1985, the year the first case of AIDS was documented in Zambia, to February 2003), 102 by-elections were held and 59 of those were due to death by disease.[x] Most of these – altogether 39 – were held between 1992 and February 2003, which are the years in which the HIV/AIDS pandemic peaked in Zambia. The majority of the deceased fell into the age range of 40-60 as illustrated in Figure 3, which is the sexually active age cohort. There were no MPs below the age of 40 at the time of the study. While there may be no specific information on the nature of the illnesses that led to the deaths of representatives, trend analyses can be indicative of the influence of the pandemic (Chirambo, 2003; 2004).

Figure 3: Age cohort and numbers of deceased MPs 1990-2003, Zambia

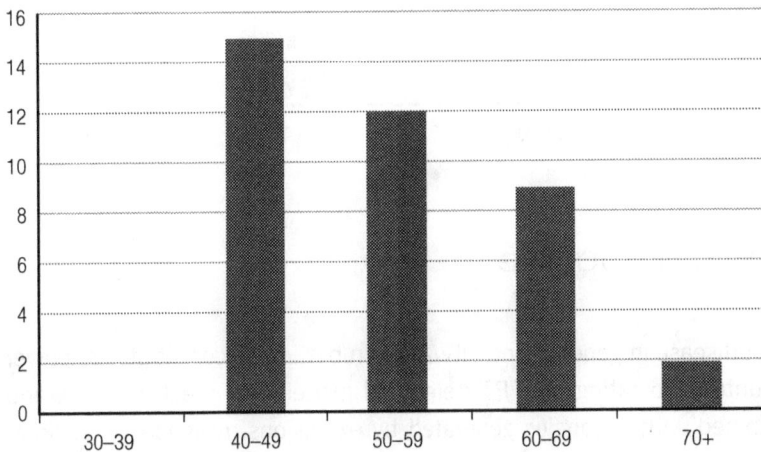

By-elections in Malawi

Our preliminary research in Malawi shows there was a steady rise in the number of legislators who died in the 1994-1995 period – which was the height of the AIDS pandemic – compared to the 1999-2004 period (Chirwa, Munthali and Mvula, 2006). Five legislators have died since the 2004 parliamentary elections.[xi]

AIDS must be one the more serious factors we consider in re-designing our electoral models because it renders some electoral systems unsustainable.

It is highly unusual for people who have a relatively higher standard of living than the general population to die in such large numbers. At a time when HIV/AIDS is the leading cause of death in Malawi – and elsewhere in sub-Saharan Africa – the trend may suggest a strong link with the pandemic, particularly since there was little or no access to ART in the early 1990s in most of Africa. Of course more research is needed to determine the ages of the MPs who died, as in the Zambia case.

Figure 4: Number of MPS deceased in Malawi, 1994-2006

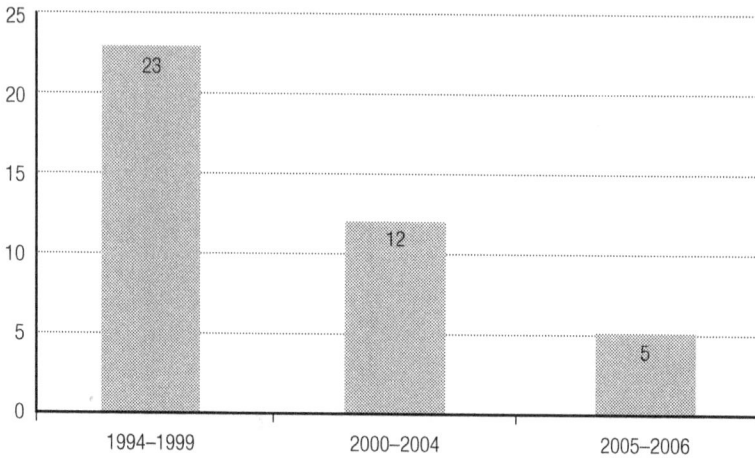

By-elections in Zimbabwe

We note that disease in general, and HIV/AIDS in particular, contributes to power shifts in countries operating the FPTP electoral model. The effect of illness and death, combined with vacancies generated by expulsions, resignations or floor-crossing by members, compelled Zimbabwe to hold 14 by-elections following the 2000 legislative polls. Eight of the by-elections arose because parliamentary representatives had died prematurely of illnesses.

Table 1: Power shifts as a result of by-elections in Zimbabwe since the 2000 general election				
Year	No of Seats			
Elections	ZANU-PF	MDC	ZANU Ndonga	Total
2000 General Election	62	57	1	120
By-Elections Since 2000*	67	52	1	120
Source: ZESN (Zimbabwe Election Support Network)				

Local government by-elections in South Africa

South Africa has also held by-elections at a local level to replace directly elected councillors. Local government by-elections in South Africa are governed by the 1998 Local Government Municipal Structures Act. Section 25 of the Act stipulates the conditions that call for a by-election:

- If the Independent Electoral Commission (IEC) does not declare the result of the local government election within a period specified in the Electoral Act;
- If a court sets aside the election of a local government structure;
- If a council is dissolved; or
- If a vacancy in a ward occurs.

The electoral system used for local government elections and by-elections is as follows: (a) for local and municipal councils (Category A and Category B respectively) 50% of ward councillors are elected directly through the FPTP system and the other 50% through the PR model in order to achieve overall political proportionality; and (b) at the district level (Category C) 40% of the councillors are directly elected by eligible district residents while 60% of the councillors are indirectly elected in that they are appointed representatives of local and municipal councils (Strand, et al, 2005).

Table 2: Local government by-elections, 2001-2004, South Africa				
Province	Size*	2001	2002	2003
Eastern Cape	601	12 (2%)	6 (1%)	12 (2%)
Free State	291	2 (0.69%)	4 (1.37%)	8 (2.75%)
Gauteng	446	9 (2.02%)	6 (1.35%)	8 (2.75%)
KwaZulu-Natal	748	27 (3.61%)	22 (2.94%)	21 (2.81%)
Limpopo	402	2 (2.24%)	5 (1.75%)	4 (1.5%)
Northern Cape	173	3 (1.73%)	9 (5.2%)	9 (5.2%)
North West	327	7 (2.14%)	8 (2.45%)	6 (1.83%)
Western Cape	340	8 (2.35%)	6 (1.76%)	9 (2.65%)
Total	3 729	79 (2.23%)	73 (1.96%)	83 (2.12%)
* Total number of ward councillors Source: Independent Electoral Commission				

In 2001, a total of 79 by-elections were held. Of these 27 were in KwaZulu-Natal and nine in Gauteng. A study undertaken by Michael Sachs (2002) provides reasons for the by-elections held by province. The fact that the number of vacancies attributed to deaths is significantly high might be indicative of a pattern we are now familiar with...possible attrition to HIV/AIDS is a strong possibility.

Table 3: By-elections per province in South Africa, 2001	
Province	Number of by-elections
KwaZulu-Natal	27
Eastern Cape	12
Gauteng	9
Mpumalanga	9
Western Cape	8
North West	7
Northern Cape	3
Free State	2
Limpopo	2
National	79
Source: Sachs, 2002	

The Sachs report indicates that of the 79 by-elections held in 2001, 34 were caused by a councillor's resignation from his or her post, 33 resulted from the death of a councillor and 12 were the result of the expulsion of a councillor either from the party or the council concerned.

Figure 5: Reasons for by-elections, 2001

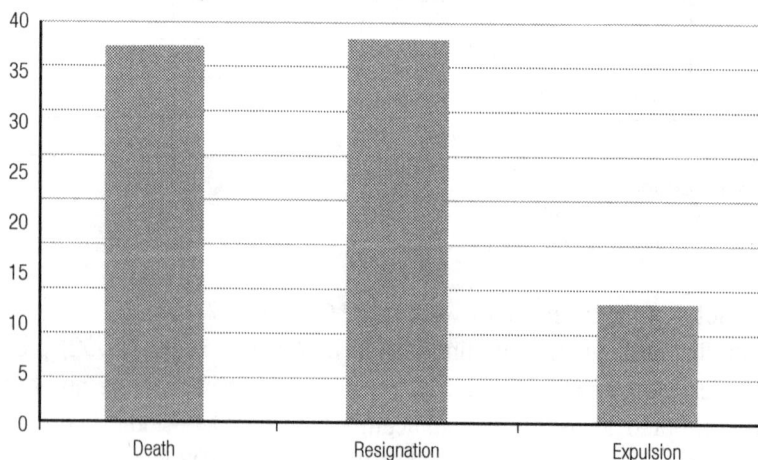

Source: Sachs, 2002

The Sachs study also found the average turn-out in by-election to be significantly lower than in general elections. He compares average turn-out in by-elections in each province with average turnout (in the same wards) in the general election in June 1999 and the municipal elections in December 2000. While the average turn-out in the December 2000 local elections was 48%, and 86% in the 1999 general elections; the study established that a comparatively lower figure of 33% of registered voters cast their ballots in the 79 local by-elections.

The significance of these data is that a proliferation of by-elections are likely to have the following effects:

- Lack of interest from voters due to known outcomes;
- Voter fatigue;
- Weaker mandates for candidates because they are elected by a minority;
- Electoral fatigue by under-resourced political parties, reducing the level of competition.

Figure 6: Comparing turn-out in by-elections with December 2000 and June 1999 polls, by province

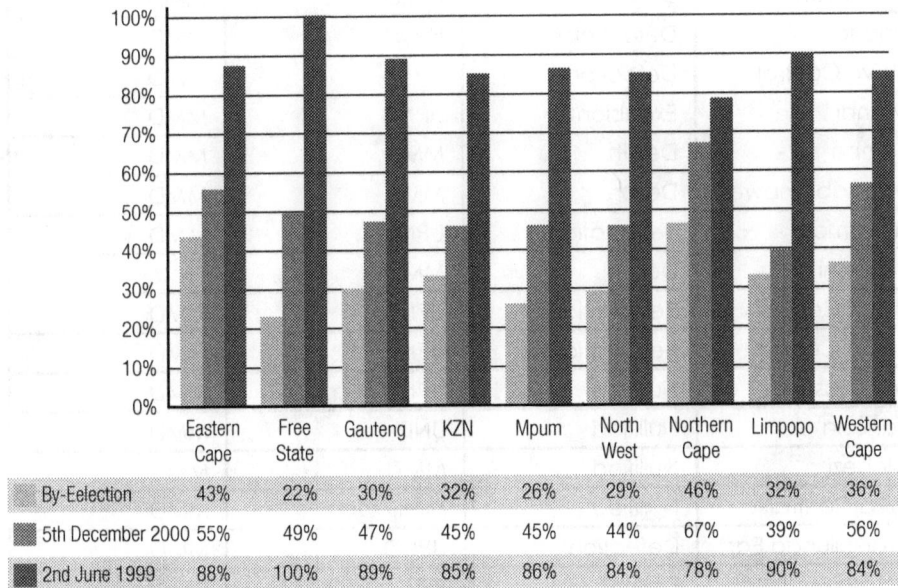

	Eastern Cape	Free State	Gauteng	KZN	Mpum	North West	Northern Cape	Limpopo	Western Cape
By-Eelection	43%	22%	30%	32%	26%	29%	46%	32%	36%
5th December 2000	55%	49%	47%	45%	45%	44%	67%	39%	56%
2nd June 1999	88%	100%	89%	85%	86%	84%	78%	90%	84%

Source: Sachs, 2002

The attrition attributable to AIDS among South Africans in the general population is itself something to seriously consider in addressing the sustainability of the electoral model at the local level.

Power shifts: altering power relations

The effect of numerous by-elections is that the opposition parties have generally lost the majority of the polls, partly perhaps due to their inability to compete with a well-resourced ruling party. In Zambia, the opposition also lost ground after entering parliament in the 2001 general elections with a combined slender majority. The 16 by-elections that followed in succession several months later were won mainly by the ruling Movement for Multi-party Democracy (MMD).

Table 4: Power shifts in parliament as a result of replacement of MPs in Zambia since the 2001 general election			
Constituency	Cause for MP replacement	Affected party	Party that gained due to replacement
Lufwanyama	Death	MMD	MMD
Bwacha	Defection	HP	MMD
Kabwe Central	Defection	HP	MMD
Mwandi	Expulsion	UPND	MMD
Keembe	Death	MMD	MMD
Mwansabombwe	Death	MMD	MMD
Nangoma	Resignation	UPND	MMD
Kantanshi	Death	MMD	PF
Solwezi Central	Resignation	UPND	MMD
Kaoma Central	Resignation	UPND	MMD
Lukulu East	Nullified	UPND	MMD
Msanzala	Nullified	UNIP	MMD
Mulobezi	Nullified	MMD	MMD
Mpika Central	Nullified	MMD	MMD
Mwaninilunga East	Defection	UPND	MMD
Kantashi	Death	PF	PF
Source: Foundation for Democratic Process (FODEP)			

Loss of representation

The immediate political cost of the death of an MP is the loss of representation by the constituency. Depending on the time it takes to replace the deceased through by-elections, this might disadvantage the masses. MPs are expected to drive development at constituency level, even though they may not always have the resources to do so. Any long absence from representation alienates the affected districts.

On the Tanzania mainland, six constituencies – Kisesa, Mbeya Vijijini, Ulanga Mashariki, Kasulu Mashariki, Rahaleo and Kilombero – had no MPs by the December 2005 general elections. Their MPs had died during the 2000-2005 parliamentary sitting. During the 1995-2000 parliament, ten MPs died (Kessy, Mallya and Mashindano, 2006).

In Malawi, it took more than a year for by-elections to be conducted in the six constituencies that fell vacant after the 2004 elections. The vacancies were attributed to a number of reasons, including deaths. The constitutional require-ment is for a by-election to be held within 90 days of the seat falling vacant (Chirwa, et al, 2006). It appears lack of funds was a constraining factor in the country's failure to hold elections timeously, Malawi being one of the poorest countries in the world.

Economic costs

There is a high cost to the Treasury in holding numerous by-elections. In December 2005 the six by-elections in Malawi cost an estimated MK65 mil-lion ($US 474 799.12), which translated into approximately MK10.8 million ($US78 889.70) per constituency (ibid).

By-elections held in Zambia have cost up to $US200 000 in the larger constituencies.[xii] In Tanzania, by-elections cost between $US300 000 and $US500 000 depending on the size of the voting district (Kessy, et al, 2006). Similarly, eight by-elections have been held in Lesotho since the country modi-fied the electoral model in 2002 from FPTP to an MMP system. Seven of the MPs had been elected through the FPTP system and one through the PR system. Each by-election cost about R1 million (roughly $US160 000.00). Three by-elections were the result of the deaths of MPs.

Although wards are smaller and therefore less costly, the cumulative effect of holding too many local by-elections can be a burden for South Africa. In our 2005 study in South Africa we were informed by the IEC that each ward by-election costs approximately R30 000. Given this estimate, the total cost for by-elections in 2001 stood at R2.3 million. This figure declined slightly to about R2.2 million in 2002, but soared to about R2.5 million in 2003. The South African local government system comprises 312 metropolitan councils, 215 dis-trict councils and 1 711 local councils. There are all in all about 3 754 wards (Strand, et al, 2005).

Impact of HIV/AIDS on electoral reform debates

The structural and strategic weaknesses provide fertile ground for a pandemic like AIDS to contribute to undermining party development.

We conclude that the List-PR system in this regard is cost-effective and is probably the best option in an HIV/AIDS-ridden environment. However, it is important to emphasise that developing an electoral system cannot be based entirely on one consideration. Countries that have employed the MMP have attempted to blend the accountability merits of the FPTP system with the inclusivity and diversity of the PR system. The indications from Lesotho suggest that the MMP system is not immune to by-elections exacerbated by premature deaths. It has been suggested during our interaction with policy-makers and researchers that the FPTP or the MMP systems could be modified to waive the use of by-elections as a mechanism for replacing leaders. Instead, the use of substitute MPs has been suggested. Senegal is an example of an MMP system that uses this model. There are a host of factors that need to be evaluated before constructing a home-grown system.

Andrew Reynolds et al (2005) spell out some criteria for electoral system design that take into account a number of important elements:

- Providing representation: That geographical representation, ideological divisions and party political situations must be taken into account in constructing an electoral system;

- Elections must be accessible and meaningful: People's votes must have a bearing on how the country is governed. Thus the choice of electoral system can influence the legitimacy of institutions;

- Facilitating stable and efficient government: The system must avoid discrimination against particular parties and interest groups; voters must perceive the system to be by and large fair;

- Providing incentives for reconciliation: Electoral systems must also serve as tools for conflict resolution within societies allowing for the inclusivity of all ethnic and interest groups to the extent possible;

- Holding the government accountable: The system must facilitate accountability, which is the bedrock of democracy;

- Encouraging political parties: The system must be seen to encourage the growth of political parties – a key factor in the consolidation of democracy;

- Promoting legislative opposition and oversight: The electoral system should assist in ushering in a viable opposition which can exercise legislative oversight over government;

- Taking into account international standards: The system must embrace international covenants, instruments and treaties affecting political issues which form the principles of free, fair and periodic elections and which advance the principle of one person, one vote;

- Making the election process sustainable: The resources of a country must be taken into account. The availability of skills and financial resources are both paramount in operating an electoral system (Reynolds, et al, 2005).

The last point reminds us of the costs illustrated above and perhaps more succinctly points out why AIDS must be one of the more serious factors we consider in re-designing our electoral models because it renders some electoral systems unsustainable.

Key findings: Impact of HIV/AIDS on electoral management and administration

The impact on EMBs has to be understood in three ways:

- The loss of internal professionals, which might affect efficiency and institutional memory;

- The loss of part-time staff who were mainly drawn from the public service's teaching profession, which compromises continuity, undermines the quality of experience and raises costs as training is then needed for new staff;

- The rapid rise in numbers of deaths renders the voters' roll unmanageable.

Our examination of various EMBs has not shown any evidence of loss of core professional staff that suggests the influence of HIV/AIDS. However, the analyses of the IEC of South Africa in 2004/5 showed that it had four staff members aged 18-24 years; 178 staff members of 25-49 years; and 28 staff members of 50-60 years. While the IEC has an internal policy on HIV/AIDS, it is clearly vulnerable to HIV/AIDS given that its core staff fell in the endangered age cohorts. The need for a strong internal policy was therefore emphasised. Studies on the impact of HIV/AIDS on parastatal/state institutional skills bases suggest that the IEC's external functions, which rely on public service workers for support during elections, are also vulnerable to the pandemic's effects. This vulnerability is aggravated by the fact that most temporary staff are from the teaching profession, which is one of the hardest hit by the HIV/AIDS pandemic. Studies by the Human Sciences Research Council (HSRC) in South Africa indicate that 4 000 teachers died in 2004 while 45 000 more, about 12.7% of the workforce, were HIV-positive. Of those who died of AIDS, 80% were under the age of 45 and 33.6% between 25 and 34. The study was conducted at 1 700 schools. Ten thousand of the 45 000 HIV-positive teachers needed ARVs (The Star, 05/04/05).

Figure 7: External impact Malawi: Causes of death among qualified teachers and staff

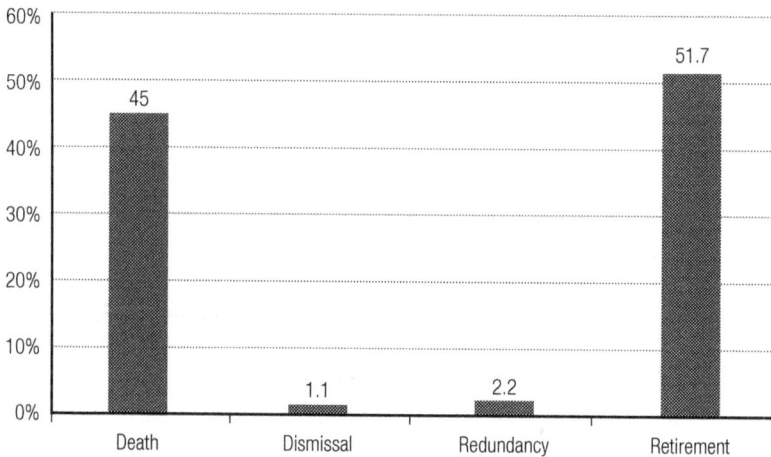

Source: Ministry of Education, 1990-2000

Michael Hendrickse, senior manager in the Electoral Democracy, Training and Legal Services Division of the IEC, explained the ramifications for his institution in our 2004/5 study:

> "An increase in the number of deceased and sick persons will have an impact on the core functions of the IEC. The delimitation of voting districts and the registration of voters will be affected as deceased persons must be taken off the voters' roll, which also affects the delimitation of voting districts as well as the arrangements for sick persons that we currently have in place. ... There will also be an impact on electoral staff especially if we cannot make use of persons who have built up electoral experience." (Interview, 2004).

In Malawi and Zambia electoral commissions also use the services of teachers extensively and there, too, the mortality among this category of workers is relatively high. A study entitled "The Impact of HIV/AIDS on the Human Resources in Malawi's Public Sector" conducted by the Malawi Institute of Management (MIM) for the government of Malawi and the UNDP illustrates a grave situation of morbidity, absenteeism and attrition due to HIV/AIDS among civil servants.

As conducting elections requires experienced staff, the vulnerability of support personnel to the disease is likely to reduce the IEC's ability to rely on them to bring their accumulated experience and skills to bear on future elections.

Key findings: Impact of HIV/AIDS on voter populations and voter registers

Voter decline in South Africa

It was established in our South Africa study that 1 488 242 of the country's registered voters died between 1999 and 2003 out of a total of 20 674 926 people who were on the voters' roll for the 2004 general elections. Deaths are concentrated in the 20-49 years and 60-79 years age groups.

We argued that the sharp increases in mortality – in some cases up to 200% – among registered voters in the 20-49 age group, particularly among women in the 30-39 years bracket, can to a large extent if not wholly be explained by AIDS.

We based our argument on the strong correspondence between the profiles that our analysis generated and those that have been described by the expert demographers in the field of HIV/AIDS. We note that it is fortunate that South Africa has citizen and voter registration systems that are compatible and equipped to timeously update the voters' roll. In this regard, the IEC of South Africa assures us that all dead voters were purged from the voters' roll before the 2004 elections, which should allay fears or perceptions of "ghost voting."

Figure 8: South Africa: Absolute and (relative) numbers of deceased voters per year

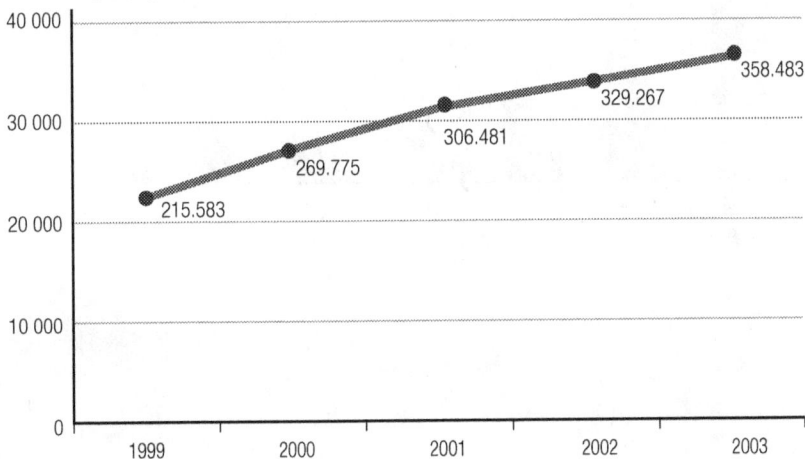

215.583
269.775
306.481
329.267
358.483

Source: IDASA

Figure 9: South Africa: Comparing mortality profiles 1999 and 2003, men, per age cohort

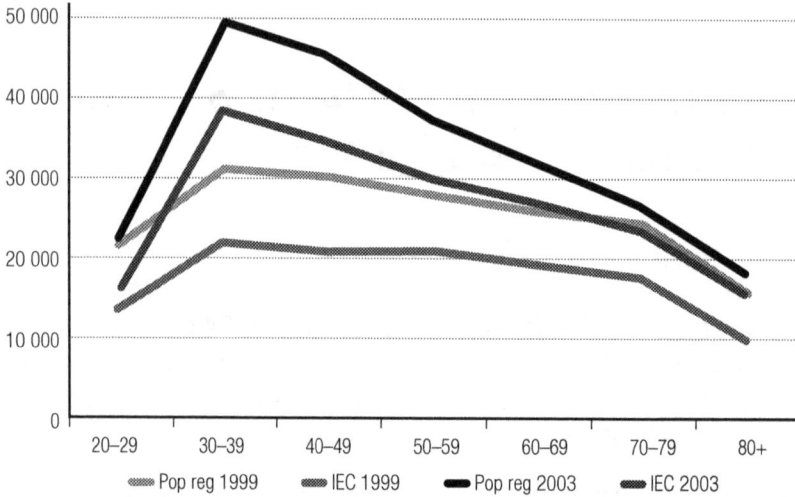

Source: IDASA

Figure 10: South Africa: Increase (in %) in relative numbers of deaths among registered voters between 1999-2003, per age and sex

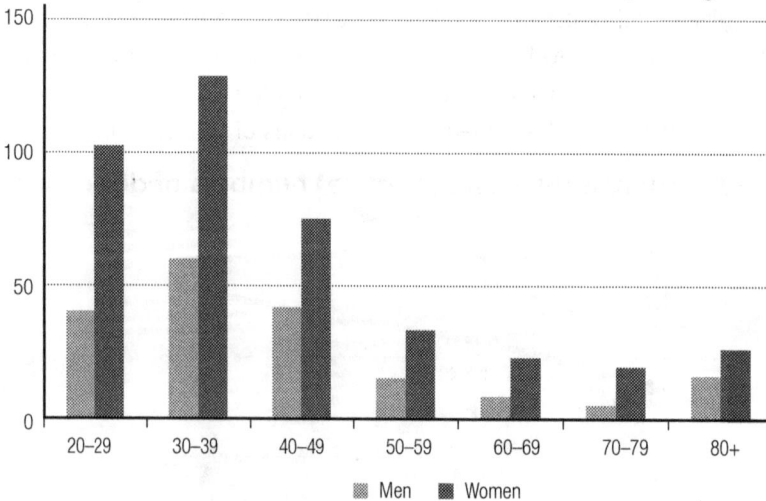

Source: IDASA

Voter decline in Zambia

Preliminary analysis of Zambia's voter profiles indicates that provinces with high HIV prevalence are the ones experiencing decline in voter pools. The country is divided into nine provinces and Table 5 shows the population size of each province from 1980 to 2000. The Copperbelt Province has the highest population followed by Lusaka, Northern, Southern and Eastern provinces. Northwestern province has the lowest population followed by Western. The data from the National Statistical Office indicates that Zambia's average annual population growth rate declined by 6.4% between 1980-1990 and 1990-2000.

There has been a decline in growth rates in all the provinces, except for Lusaka, Northern and Luapula provinces. The lowest population growth rate has been that of Copperbelt province, which declined from 1.5% in the 1980-1990 intercensal period to 1.3% in the 1990-2000 intercensal period. The highest population growth rates have been in Northern (4.3%), Lusaka (3.8%), North-Western (3.4%) and Luapula provinces (3.4%). It is estimated that more than 650 000 Zambians have died from the pandemic. If current trends continue 1.6 million more may die before the year 2015 (Tapfumaneyi, 2003). The prevalence of HIV infection in the urban areas of Zambia is 28% and 14% in rural areas in the 15 to 49-year-old age group. HIV prevalence in the whole country was reported at 21.5% by UNAIDS. At the time of the study, HIV prevalence was twice as high in urban areas than in rural areas (ibid).

Table 5: Population size by province, Zambia				
Province	1980	1990	2000	Prevalence rate
Central	511 905	771 819	1 006 766	18.7%
Copperbelt	1 257 178	1 458 471	1 657 646	26.3%
Eastern	650 902	1 004 700	1 300 973	16.5%
Luapula	420 966	564 490	784 613	16.2%
Lusaka	691 054	991 230	1 432 401	27.3%
Northern	674 750	925 388	1 407 088	13.5%
North/Western	302 668	438 215	610 975	11.7%
Southern	671 923	965 593	1 302 660	15.7%
Western	486 455	638 761	782 509	18.9%
Total	5 661 801	7 759 167	10 285 631	
Source: Population and Demography Branch Central Statistics				

Although Zambia recorded its highest voter participation rates in the 2001 presidential elections, an estimated 67%, the statistics raise a number of questions when we consider the absolute figures of registered and actual voters since the first multi-party polls in 1991 (see Table 6). Despite the increase in the number of eligible voters, the number of registered voters has continued to decline. The total number of voters has also declined in absolute terms between the 1991 and 2001 elections.

Table 6: Voter registration and actual votes in Zambian elections 1991-2001

Year	Eligible Voters	Registered Voters	Reg/ Eligible	Total Vote	Vote/Reg.	Vote/ Elig Vote
1991	3.8 mill	2.93 mill	77%	1.31 mill	45%	35%
1996	4.4 mill	2.26 mill	51%	1.26 mill	55%	30%
2001	4.68 mill	2.6 mill	55%	1.7 mill	67%	37%

Source: Adapted from Rakner and Svåsand (2003)

Without taking into account the absolute numbers of voters who were eligible to vote and the total figures of registered voters and actual voters, the 12% increase in turnout between the 1996 and 2001 polls could be misleading. Stakeholders interviewed in a study on the impact of donor funding on Zambia's tripartite presidential, parliamentary and local government elections of 2001 (Chirambo, Nel and Erasmus, 2003) highlighted a number of factors to explain comparatively lower registration in 2001, which included long distances to registration centres, disillusionment with politics, poor publicity campaigns and an over-elaborate registration process which discouraged potential electors (Chirambo, et al, 2003). HIV/AIDS was not cited as a possible explanation for the comparatively lower numbers.

The loss of a patron can spell the end of a political party.

Preliminary studies have shown however that of the country's nine provinces, Lusaka with an HIV prevalence of 27.3%, Copperbelt 26.3% and Western 18.9% have shown the sharpest decline. The Copperbelt province, the mining region of the country, has seen its voter population decline by 149 349 (602 589 in 1991 to 453 240 in 2001) (Tapfumaneyi, 2003).

One of the strongest explanations for the drop could be the mass unemployment leading to labour migration that arose from the privatisation of the mining and manufacturing industries on the Copperbelt. It is possible that skilled labour moved to other towns, cities and neighbouring countries as the job market shrank (Tapfumaneyi, 2003; Chirambo, 2004). An on-going study by IDASA expects to unravel this phenomenon further.

Voter decline in Malawi

In 2003, a commissioner of the Malawi Electoral Commission (MEC) said at the AIDS and Governance Forum held in Cape Town that EMBs in the region were aware of the complications HIV/AIDS posed for electoral management and administration but had not given them enough attention for unexplained reasons:

> *"The impact of HIV/AIDS has forced electoral management bodies to face a number of problems regarding the voters' roll. The number of registered voters on the voters roll is not a true reflection of what is on the ground. Our voters' rolls are bloated with dead voters"* (Chirambo and Caesar, 2003: 28).

The commissioner was speaking in her capacity as a representative of the SADC-ECF. Chirwa, et al (2006) point out that the component of the electoral system most susceptible to the impact of the HIV/AIDS epidemic in Malawi is the voters' roll and its mismanagement. Malawi's voters' roll is not regularly updated. The researchers describe this phenomenon in greater detail:

> *"The only system of updating the roll is the fresh registration at the beginning of a fresh election. The database on which the voters' roll is based is not entirely credible. The absence of a civic register means that there is no system of reporting births and deaths, hence the country's demographic database tends to be outdated. The voters' roll thus inherently creates political tensions, especially at the time of the announcement of elections. This tension arises from the fact that the exact size of Malawi's voters' roll remains unknown. The effects of the HIV/AIDS pandemic on the country's demographic database compounds these tensions. With deaths not being timely reported and the roll not being timely purged of the dead voters, there is a real risk that the roll is bloated with dead people."*

In 1999, a total of 5 071 822 voters were registered and of these 2 417 713 were registered in the southern region, 1 975 203 in the central region and 678 906 in the northern region. However in April 2004, the MEC announced that 6 668 839 voters had registered for the May 18, 2004 presidential and parliamentary elections.[xiii] These figures were challenged by opposition political parties and other institutions with the National Statistical Office taking the lead. It described the figure as "bogus" because it did not conform to the country's natural demographic trends.

The result of Malawi's problematic voters' roll is a weak mandate for the new government and post-election conflict over outcomes. Malawi has been preoccupied with impeachment tensions since the last presidential polls.

Key findings: Impact of HIV/AIDS on political parties

Political parties have flourished under the new democratic dispensation in Africa. Emergent political parties, bolstered by relaxed registration rules, have made important contributions to "good" governance and democratic accountability, allowing for diverse interests to emerge.

Studies by the United Nations Economic Commission for Africa (UNECA) indicate that Chad has 73 political parties, South Africa 140, Mali 91, Ethiopia 79, Burkina Faso 47, Morocco Nigeria and Botswana each have 30, Egypt 17 and Ghana 10 (UNECA, 2005). The viability of these political parties varies from country to country. In fact, the party system is yet to fully develop on the continent. Most political parties are headed by patrons who not only finance the institutions but also provide the leadership. Political parties are formed usually before a major poll and dissipate upon failure to access power (UNECA, 2005).

Discrimination is the exclusion that follows stigmatisation and can be institutional in character.

In Malawi, of the nine parties that won parliamentary seats in the 2004 election, only three were more than ten years old. These were the Malawi Congress Party, the Alliance for Democracy and the United Democratic Front. The rest were created within three years of the election (Chirwa, et al, 2006). In Zambia, nearly all the opposition parties that contested the second multi-party election in 1996 had collapsed by the time the country held its third election in 2001, except for the United National Independence Party (UNIP) the former ruling party, and it in fact boycotted the poll (SARDC, 2005).

South Africa, with a PR electoral system at national level and state financing for political parties, has a relatively stable party environment as there seems to be an incentive to exist beyond elections. In most other countries, except for ruling parties which tend to have access to state resources, opposition elements lack organisational strength, are administratively weak and poor on ideology and mandate. Political parties also lack internal democracy compromising the smooth alternation of power.

Implications for party structures

The structural and strategic weaknesses provide fertile ground for a pandemic like AIDS, to contribute to undermining party development. There are three levels at which HIV/AIDS will impact on political party structures:

- Organisational: The loss of cadres and members affects electioneering capacity;

- Financial: Loss of members reduces subscriptions;

- Leadership: The loss of a patron spells the end of a party or compromises electoral viability and financial status.

The single common feature emerging from preliminary research on political parties in several of the six countries being studied is the poor record-keeping amongst the entities. Membership cards are often distributed without charge; therefore using a decline in subscription as a proxy indicator for member attrition is futile. However perceptions of loss to HIV/AIDS amongst members are acknowledged in Zambia and South Africa by party and government officials alike.

"It is now an acknowledged fact that political parties, which are an essential part of any multi-party democracy, are affected by HIV/AIDS. Almost all political parties in this country have been losing leaders at various levels due to HIV/AIDS-related illness and deaths."[xiv]

In our 2005 study, the leading political parties in South Africa, including the African National Congress (ANC), the Democratic Alliance (DA) and the Inkatha Freedom Party (IFP), did acknowledge that HIV/AIDS does or could strain party structures, creating an increased need to replace cadres who have succumbed to illness, especially HIV/AIDS. Although no discernible functional defects have arisen in the party structures, a loss of seniority and experience was reported. A more direct impact acknowledged by religious-based parties, such as the African Christian Democratic Party (ACDP), is the time HIV/AIDS-related deaths have tended to commit political leaders to in terms of officiating at recurrent funerals of cadres. This might affect their organisational capacities.

Malawi provides some empirical data on attrition in the structures of its founding party, the Malawi Congress Party (MCP). Chirwa, et al (2006) indicate that confidential correspondence shows that the party lost at least 22 members of its district committees, at least 13 members of its regional committees and not fewer than eight members of its central executive committee between 1987 and 1993.

"These figures are drawn from letters between the district officials and the national executive. The records are not comprehensive, and the causes of the deaths are not stated. It cannot therefore be assumed or concluded that these were all AIDS-related deaths. What is known, for sure, is that by this time the effects of AIDS had started to be felt in the country, after its first reported case in 1985. Of the 22 deaths at the district level, 19 occurred

between 1990 and 1993; and of the 13 at the regional level, 11 occurred during the same period; and all the eight at the national executive level occurred during the same period. This pattern suggests a connection with the felt effects of the pandemic at this time" (Chirwa, et al; 2006).

Key findings: Impact of HIV/AIDS on political participation

Stigma and discrimination: AIDS as a political weapon

UNAIDS defines stigmatisation as "a process of devaluation within a particular culture or setting where attitudes are seized upon and defined as discredible or not worthy" (Panos/Unicef, 2004). Essentially this means a group of people are cast aside based on the assumption that they are different or apart from the normal social order. It connotes a sense of shame arising from the apparent violation of a set of values or norms by an individual or group. Discrimination is the exclusion that follows this process and can be institutional in character.

A salient feature noted in our research in Zambia is the use of HIV/AIDS as a weapon in electoral politics. Candidates who are perceived to be sick are de-campaigned and destroyed before the eyes of the electorate. Weight loss is closely associated with AIDS and has caused opposition parties to cast doubt on the health of leading candidates and incumbents alike. In our post-research stakeholder meetings with the ruling MMD and opposition parties in July 2006 in Zambia this was further underlined by top party officials.

In a discussion with ruling and opposition parties in Zambia all of the parties present stated categorically that they would not put forward an HIV-positive candidate for fear of him or her being rejected by the electorate. They also saw such candidates as liabilities who were likely to cost their parties precious parliamentary seats through losing by-elections. These fears appear to be accentuated by public demands for all political candidates to be tested for HIV/AIDS, a debate that permeated Zambian society in the run-up to the 2006 presidential elections (Simutanyi and Rubvuta, 2006).

The debate on Voluntary Counselling and Testing (VCT) for elected representatives has also engulfed Namibia. Former Swapo MP, Ben Ulenga, who was Deputy Minister of Local Government at the time, stirred a heated debate when he announced his intention in 1996 to take a test for HIV. He also alleged that half the national parliament was infected by the virus. His negative results did not inspire others to follow suit (Hopwood, Hunter and Kellner; 2006). In the three countries being studied that have released preliminary results, there is not a single elected member or cabinet minister known to be HIV-positive. This contradicts the statistics. There seem to be deep-rooted fears among the political elite to expose their medical records in the event that they are sero-positive. This suggests a denialism that complicates the fight against stigma and discrimination in the lower echelons of society, and for that matter in electoral politics.

AIDS sickness has been highlighted in Tanzania, Zambia, Namibia and South Africa as an impediment to political participation.

The message from the political elite is that HIV/AIDS is a disease of the poor and unless it translates into votes it will not form part of a mainstream leadership agenda. AIDS, it seems, still carries a lot of stigma; it is to be feared and used only as an offensive weapon in the theatre of politics. Accusations by Ugandan President Yoweri Museveni reported in the New York Times in March 2001 underline this point. He denounced his main political rival, Kizza Besigye, as an AIDS patient. Besigye, brushing off the allegations, responded by rallying infected and affected people and accusing Museveni of discriminating against the sick.

Suggestions have been made by PLWHAs in Tanzania to promote the idea of creating a special seat in parliament for people with HIV/AIDS so that a more authoritative figure could champion the fight within the institution. It is felt that such a move might provide a new form of leadership around the disease based on experience. But given the reluctance of leaders across the region to present their medical records, there is little indication of MPs heading to VCT centres any time soon.

Stigma, discrimination as impediments to citizen participation

AIDS sickness has been highlighted in Tanzania, Zambia, Namibia and South Africa as an impediment to political participation. Although the levels of stigma differ from country to country, it was only in South Africa that PLWHAs expressed fears about their status compromising their engagement with the wider public in an election. We can explain this by appreciating the mature nature of the epidemic in these countries. In our South African study, stigma and discrimination resonated as the single most dominant determinants for lack of participation in elections by PLWHAs and care-givers in rural KwaZulu Natal. Focus group discussions with PLWHAs and care-givers who were all registered voters for the 2004 election, held in urban and rural areas of KwaZulu-Natal, yielded seemingly well-founded fears that communities will further ostracise or marginalise those infected and affected if they appeared at major public events. The participants' opinions correlate with the findings of studies on stigma and discrimination, particularly the South African Department of Health study of 2002, that HIV/AIDS remains a taboo topic among some South African communities, especially in the rural enclaves. The sense of stigma, it seems, is strongest where people are symptomatic; participants said that most members of the communities would not stand in the same queue with someone with visible signs of disease e.g. body rashes or sores. Based on these discussions, we concluded that in South Africa people who have visible signs of HIV/AIDS and those who have publicly declared their status are more likely to withdraw from publicly voting, particularly if they are located in a rural area.

There is nothing to suggest that PLWHAs have lost the will to participate in political life. In fact, the majority of participants expressed a desire to participate but said they were constrained by attitudinal and structural factors. Structural factors included lack of transport, toilets, seating facilities and running water at polling stations. These results are not representative of the opinions of all PLWHAs as only 68 people participated in the focus groups, but they are indicative of such attitudes and may have external validity.

Special votes

South Africa operates a special vote mechanism to assist the disabled, business people and travellers to vote from home or by post if they are not able to present themselves on election day due to commitments or ailments. It is acknowledged that the "special vote" is a very useful institutional arrangement to ensure, as far as possible, that people are not disenfranchised by being disabled, pregnant or by virtue of attending to business or educational trips abroad (Lodge, 2004; EISA, 2004). More than 650 000 voters used this special vote in the 2004 election but records do not indicate the reasons advanced by applicants for using it. Hence, we cannot determine to what extent people with AIDS-related complexes used this facility, if at all.

While this instrument may be a possible solution to encourage the participation of PLWHAs in elections, people with HIV/AIDS in Tanzania and Zambia have strongly dismissed this as a potential source of discrimination. The dominant view is that any special mechanisms tailored for PLWHAs would isolate them and expose them to further scorn. This argument suggests that other creative modes of voting, including the use of mobile polling stations as in Namibia, could facilitate voting by hospital-ridden patients and those constrained by physical demands and time constraints.

Public opinion

More detailed analyses of Afrobarometer public opinion data from Southern African countries (including South Africa) in our 2005 study suggest an increase in public awareness of HIV/AIDS as a political and social problem. There is, however, no basis to argue that HIV/AIDS is shaping public opinion in a consistent fashion across the Southern African region. South Africa is an exception as statistical patterns indicate that people who suffer personal loss are more likely to prioritise HIV/AIDS in their demands for government interventions. Nevertheless there is nothing to suggest at this point that people affected by HIV/AIDS would change their choice of political party as a result of this disaffection. Studies by the Afrobarometer survey released in 2006 show that HIV/AIDS ranks among the top five priorities for South Africans, along with unemployment, housing, crime and poverty. The study involved a representative sample of 2 400 South Africans and it was conducted in January and February 2006 by Citizen Surveys.

Figure 11: South African's public agenda, 2006

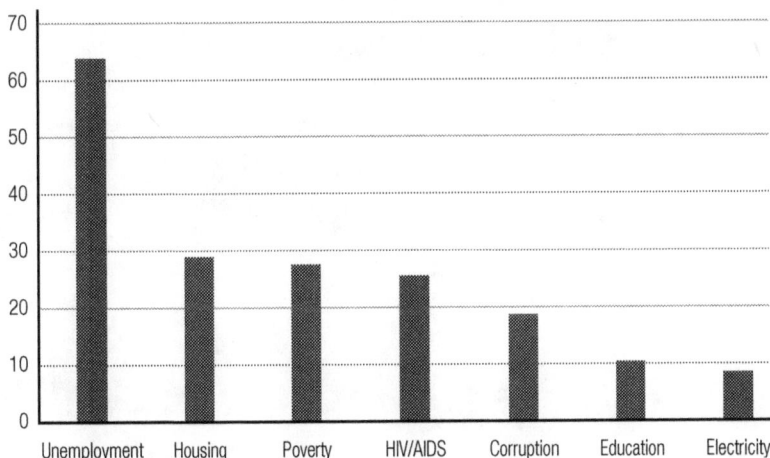

Source: Afrobarometer, 2006

"I was sick and I could not walk".
Registered voter, rural African male, 18-24, Nongoma, South Africa.

Activism by social movements such as the Treatment Action Campaign (TAC) continues to raise awareness of government responsibilities on HIV/AIDS and are likely to raise the status of the pandemic on the national priority list as society comes to understand the full impacts of the pandemic. This will pose further governance challenges to government on the quality of delivery in the health sector in general and on HIV/AIDS in particular.

Conclusions

Our ongoing research continues to unravel a complex interaction between politics and AIDS. The challenge for researchers in this field is to explore alternative avenues in which to frame the response to AIDS. There are a number of issues that arise from our pilot project, our South African report and the preliminary multi-country studies which suggest that we cannot do business the way it has been done over the years. Certainly, new radical strategies need to be adopted to break the back of stigma and that call for fresh approaches to sensitising leaders and citizens. Challenging the institutional aspects of discrimination which manifest at state and employer level and in financial institutions which often deny applicants cover and loans if they are positive might be one way of rendering AIDS a "normal" disease. As matters stand, the fear exhibited among the political elite and citizens alike indicate that VCT and ART alone are not an adequate incentive for testing. The loss of economic and political benefits is a side-effect of VCT that commands a level of fear that leads to denial and unresponsiveness to campaigns for openness. There are of course some immediate political steps that can be taken to help absorb the economic and political shocks attributed to AIDS, particularly because electoral reform debates in most SADC countries have been ongoing:

1. Clearly, the FPTP system needs revisiting. It fails to meet the single key condition that is emphasised in this research, namely sustainability. It is suggested that modification be sought to do away with by-elections. Arguments may be raised about the loss of a competitive edge to this system should by-elections be eliminated, but while a wholesale departure from FPTP to PR is the easy route to take, the concerns around accountability or lack of it raised by many experts and interest groups cannot be ignored. The MMP system incorporates the strengths of both systems but is itself vulnerable to the pandemic unless adjustments are made – again to eliminate the requirement for by-elections. As SADC countries embark upon electoral reforms, issues around HIV/AIDS should be taken on board in the determination of the appropriate electoral systems to be adopted.

2. There is an immense problem in addressing AIDS-related stigma and discrimination; the fact that it now emerges in the political arena as a "weapon" undermines the role of leadership in dealing with it. Activists and experts alike need to address the real fears surrounding HIV/AIDS, which are institutional in character, including citizens' fear that they could lose access to economic goods should they be found positive. Also, the fact that a positive status can cost political careers also needs to be addressed.

3. It is clear from preliminary reports in the multi-country study that we are unlikely to witness elected political leaders disclosing their HIV sero-positive status anytime soon. Obviously such disclosure could serve to present HIV as a "normal" infection, one that does not render the infected individual unworthy of engaging in politics or official duties. Such action could win many battles against stigma. Given the unrealistic prospect of this happening, we should perhaps consider the suggestion of creating a special seat for PLWHAs in decision-making mechanisms.

4. The research suggests further that there are roles for the EMBs in the HIV/AIDS field. The impact of stigma on participation, though only indicative in rural South Africa, deserves attention as it may be more extensive than this study suggests, with ramifications for the involvement of individuals infected and affected in politics. EMBs could assist by incorporating non-discriminatory messages in their voter education campaigns which encourage more people to participate and be tolerant. Only the Zanzibar Electoral Commission used AIDS messages during the 2005 election in Tanzania. However, this is a role to be championed by political leaders themselves, who ultimately are the beneficiaries of power in government.

Formation of bi-partisan coalitions

There might be a need to establish a strategic bi-partisan extra-parliamentary body that involves all elected national representatives. Tanzania, for instance, has established the Tanzania Parliamentarians AIDS Coalition (TAPAC) whose membership is open to former and serving MPs from all parties. TAPAC has empowered MPs; enabled interaction with constituencies and AIDS bodies; and facilitated strong leadership at parliamentary level while maintaining HIV/AIDS on the agenda in parliamentary committees. As nearly all MPs are members of TAPAC, this setup provides a good example of a practical way of de-politicising HIV/AIDS while dealing with issues such as stigma and discrimination. However, such coalitions will probably only work in certain political environments. They are unlikely to function in polarised situations.

Treatment vs. worst case scenarios

Many affected African countries have invested in mass treatment programmes. Even though the resources do not match the crisis, there is an all-round effort to mitigate the impact of the pandemic. South Africa has launched possibly the largest treatment programme in the world. Although the mechanics of it have yet to be lubricated, there is the potential for this programme to contribute significantly to efforts to reduce HIV/AIDS-related stigma and discrimination. The sooner the pandemic is seen less as a death sentence than a chronic illness the better for the communities that constantly ostracise PLWHAs for fear of contagion.

Figure 12: People receiving therapy (thousands)

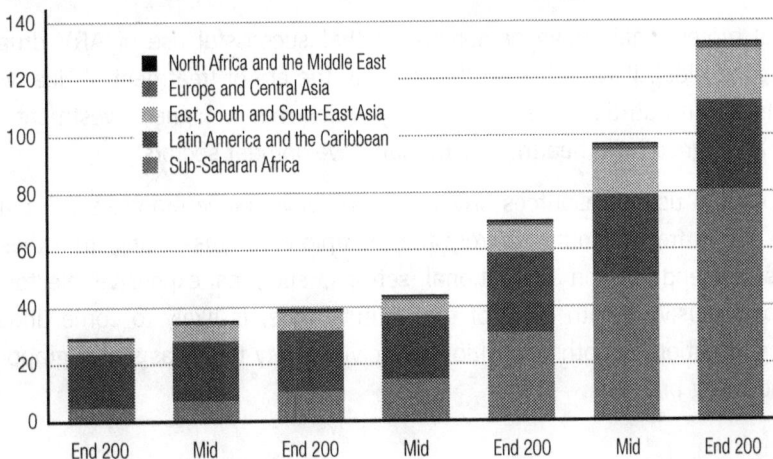

Source: WHO/UNAIDS, 2005

It should also be considered, however, that treatment by itself does not guarantee a reversal of the multi-facetted impacts of the pandemic. The operational efficiency and capacity of health systems to deliver, along with food security and nutrition strategies will ultimately determine how effectively the pandemic is dealt with in the next 20 years. It is critical to mention that despite all the publicity about treatment, coverage in sub-Saharan Africa remains limited.

AIDS, it must be remembered, is also depleting skills in the health sector. In addition, Africa is losing 23 000 health professionals annually to the West where they get better packages and working conditions (Nepad, 2003).

Worryingly, a third of sub-Saharan Africans, about 200 million people, are reported to be chronically malnourished. Experts say malnutrition is a consequence of poverty, disease and mortality. More than half the deaths of children under the age of five and almost 60% of all malaria deaths are attributed to malnutrition.

"For the 25 million people in Africa living with HIV/AIDS, malnutrition and disease lock in a vicious negative cycle, HIV compromises nutritional status and increases susceptibility to infection while malnutrition weakens immunity, worsens the severity of infections and hastens the onset of disease" (Nepad, 2005).

The underlying causes of disease, according to the Nepad report, are food insecurity; inadequate care and feeding practices; limited access to health services, clean portable water and sanitation; and other environmental factors. Nepad experts assert that the basic causes are located in the issues of governance, peace and security, as well as global factors, for example global agricultural policies which disadvantage African producers.

Medical professionals have demonstrated that successful use of ARV drugs requires good diets. It would seem that even in the era of treatment, Africa will need to focus on nutrition and food security which means higher investment in the food and agriculture, health, and human development sectors.

The optimum use of resources driven by good governance practices will play a critical role in freeing countries from the multiple problems arising from these scenarios. Expenditure on institutional set-ups, such as expensive electoral models or exclusive health care for the political elite, is likely to come under increasing attention by both opposition and civil society forces as states grapple with contending priorities.

Bibliography

Afrobarometer Briefings, (2006), 7 June.

Barnett, T. and Whiteside, A. (2002), *AIDS in the Twenty-First Century: Disease and Globalisation*. New York: Palgrave Macmillan.

Cheema, G.S. (2000), *Good Governance: A Path to Poverty Eradication*. New York: UNDP.

Chirambo, K. (2003), "Impact of HIV/AIDS on Electoral Processes in Southern Africa". Presentation to the UNDP/IDASA Satellite Conference, Nairobi, September.

Chirambo, K. (2004), *AIDS and Electoral Democracy: Implications for Participation, Political Stability and Accountability in Southern Africa*, Johannesburg: EISA.

Chirambo, K. (2005), *AIDS & Electoral Democracy: Insights into Impacts on Africa's Democratic Institutions*. Cape Town: IDASA.

Chirambo, K. and Caesar, M. (eds.) (2003), *HIV/AIDS and Governance in Southern Africa: Emerging Theories and Perspectives*. Cape Town: IDASA.

Chirambo, K., Nel, N. and Erasmus, C. (2003), *Zambia Presidential, Parliamentary and Local Government Elections, 2001: Evaluation of Impact of Donor Investment*. Cape Town: IDASA.

CHGA (2004), *Q & A on HIV/AIDS and Governance in Africa*. Addis Ababa: Commission for HIV/AIDS Governance in Africa/Economic Commission for Africa.

Chirwa, W., Munthali, A. and Mvula, P. (forthcoming), "HIV/AIDS and Democratic Governance in Malawi: Illustrating the Impact on Electoral Processes", Cape Town: IDASA (preliminary report).

EISA (1999), *Comparative Political Parties Funding Practices*. Johannesburg: EISA.

EISA (2003), *Principles for Election Management, Monitoring and Observation in the SADC Region*. Johannesburg: Electoral Commissions Forum/EISA.

Hopwood, G., Hunter, J. and Kellner, D. (forthcoming), "HIV/AIDS and Democratic Governance in Namibia: Illustrating the Impact on Electoral Processes", Cape Town: IDASA. (preliminary report).

HSRC (2002), *Nelson Mandela/HSRC Study on HIV/AIDS*. Cape Town: HSRC.

IDASA/HEARD/DARU (2002), AIDS and Democracy Workshop for Researchers Report.

Kessy, F., Mallya, E. and Masindano, O. (forthcoming), "HIV/AIDS and Democratic

Governance in Tanzania: Illustrating the Impact on Electoral Processes", Cape Town: IDASA (preliminary report).

Lodge. T. (2004), *Handbook of South African Electoral Laws and Regulations.* Johannesburg: EISA.

Matlosa, K. (2003), "Electoral System Reform, Democracy and Stability in the SADC Region", Johannesburg: EISA, Research Report No 1.

Mattes, R. (2003), "Institutional Mandates and the Challenges of HIV and AIDS on Democracy in Southern Africa", Pretoria: Institute for Security Studies.

Mattes, R. (2003), "Healthy Democracies? Potential Impact of HIV/AIDS on Democracy in Southern Africa", in Chirambo, K. and Caesar, M. (eds.) *AIDS and Governance in Southern Africa: Emerging Theories and Perspectives.* Cape Town: IDASA.

National Intelligence Council (2005), "Mapping Sub-Saharan Africa's Future", Conference Report.

Mail & Guardian (2004). "AIDS High on Malawi Poll Agenda", May 21-27.

Nepad (2003). *NEPAD Health Strategy.* Pretoria: Nepad.

Nepad (2005), *Focus on Africa*, issue 104, August.

New York Times (2001), "AIDS Permeates Uganda Politics Too", March 12, Ian Fisher.

Rakner, L. and Svåsand, L. (2003), "The Quality of Electoral Processes: Zambian Election 1991 – 2001", *African Social Research*, Vol. 2000/2001, Nos 45/46, pp. 1-23.

Panos/Unicef (2004). "Stigma, HIV/AIDS and Prevention of Mother-to Child Transmission: A Pilot Study in Zambia, Ukraine, India and Burkina Faso", London: Panos/Unicef.

Reynolds, A., Reilly, B. and Ellis, A., with Cheibub, J.A. (2005), *Electoral System Design: The New International IDEA Handbook.* Stockholm: IDEA

Sachs M. (2002), "By Elections in 2001: A Statistical Review", in UMRABULO. No 14, April, also available at www.anc.org.za/ancdocs/pubs/umrabulo/umrabulo14/elections.html

SARDC (2005), *Zambia Democracy Fact File.* Harare: SARDC.

Schonteich, M. (2003a), "Impact and Mainstreaming of HIV and AIDS within Security Institutions," Pretoria: Institute for Security Studies.

Schonteich, M. (2003b), "The Impact and Mainstreaming of HIV and AIDS within Security Institutions", in Chirambo, K. and Caesar, M. (eds.) *HIV/AIDS and*

Governance in Southern Africa: Emerging Theories and Perspectives. Cape Town: IDASA.

Simbao, K. (2005), Opening speech at the IDASA/FODEP/INESOR Policy Forum on AIDS and Elections quoted in Chirambo, K. (2005), *AIDS & Electoral Democracy: Insights into Impacts on Africa's Democratic Institutions.* Cape Town: IDASA.

Simutanyi, N. and Rubvuta, E. (forthcoming), "HIV/AIDS and Democratic Governance in Zambia: Illustrating the Impact on Electoral Processes", Cape Town: IDASA.

Star (2005), "11 Teachers a Day Die of AIDS", April 1. Ndivhuwo Khangale & Sapa.

Strand, P., Matlosa, K., Strode, A. and Chirambo, K. (2005), *HIV/AIDS and Democratic Governance in South Africa: Illustrating the Impact on Electoral Processes.* Cape Town: IDASA.

Tapfumaneyi, W.O. (2003), *Zambia Status Report.* Pretoria: IDASA.

UNAIDS (2003). *Epidemiological Update.* Geneva: UNAIDS.

UNDP (1997), "Reconceptualizing Governance", New York: UNDP, Discussion Paper 2.

UNDP (2002), "Deepening Democracy in a Fragmented World," Human Development Report 2002, New York: UNDP, also available at www.undp.org

UNECA (2005), *Striving for Good Governance in Africa.* Addis Ababa: United Nations Economic Commission for Africa.

Youde, J. (2001), *All the Voters Will be Dead: HIV/AIDS and Democratic Legitimacy and Stability in Africa.* University of Iowa.

WHO/UNAIDS (2005), "Progress on global access to HIV antiretroviral therapy: An update on '3 by 5'", WHO/UNAIDS.

Endnotes

i   Research shows that Proportional Representation (PR) systems maximise the potential for gender and ethnic diversity, therefore minimising conflict and fostering inclusivity in policy decisions. Plurality majority systems, such as First-Past-the-Post (FPTP), generally fail to achieve these ends; the competitive nature of the system does not favour disadvantaged groups such as women and ethnic minorities. The electoral systems will also determine the nature of political party development. PR systems will generate policy-based parties because they have to appeal to the entire population to garner a decent proportion of the national vote. In FPTP, studies have shown that the opposite is true; political parties can be personality-based, without clear policy and ideological direction, but still claim a presence at constituency level.

ii   Barnett and Whiteside explain that the epidemic comes in successive waves, the first being HIV infection followed several years later by a wave of opportunistic infections and finally a third wave of illness and death.

iii   Mattes refers to the work of Larry Diamond and Richard Joseph in addition to Freedom House, a US research institute. Democracies are categorised as follows:
   • Liberal or 'free' democracies: countries that combine genuine political competition with a full range of political freedoms and civil rights. South Africa, Namibia and Botswana fall in this category but an identifiable weakness is that they all have dominant power structures that limit effective competition. They risk being semi-democratic as a result.
   • Electoral democracies: countries that combine genuine political competition with an insufficient protection of rights. Malawi, Tanzania, Mozambique and Lesotho are rated as 'partly free' by Freedom House, thus falling into this category.
   • Pseudo or virtual democracies: These countries hold elections and allow opposition parties, but competition, pluralism and rights of association, speech and media are actively constrained by the state. Zambia and Zimbabwe are rated as 'partly free' by Freedom House but score sufficiently badly on political rights that they fall into the 'pseudo-democracy' category. Mattes adds that US research institute Freedom House ratings show retrograde trends in political freedom and civil liberties in Malawi and Zimbabwe.

iv   In his paper at IDASA's Governance and AIDS Forum in 2003, Schonteich speculated that "a large influx of orphaned children into urban slums surrounding most larger Southern African cities will exacerbate socio-economic conditions, thereby creating a vibrant breeding ground for a variety of social ills such as crime".

v   Proceedings of HEARD/IDASA/DARU Workshop on Democracy and AIDS in Southern Africa: Setting the Research Agenda, Cape Town, 22-23 April 2002.

vi   The SADC comprises Angola, Botswana, Lesotho, Namibia, Malawi, Mauritius, Tanzania, Seychelles, South Africa, Swaziland, Zambia and Zimbabwe. No authoritative study has explained the differences in the patterns of infection between west and southern Africa.

vii   Cheema, (2000) defines governance as "a set of values, policies and institutions by which a society manages its economic, political and social processes at all levels through interaction among government, civil society and the private sector".

viii   Counter-arguments hold that democracies can be encumbered by a paralysis of governance when consensus is not reached because of the often elaborate consultative decision-making processes. The emergency context of HIV/AIDS requires decisive action, which may even compromise the rights of the infected in the interest of the unaffected, if only to isolate and contain the pandemic. Authoritarian states such as Thailand, Cuba and Uganda have fared better in stemming the tide of infections while emergent democracies of a similar profile have tended to struggle. In essence, the political discourse on AIDS remained very much a theoretical enterprise.

ix   Preliminary findings of IDASA s multi-country study, forthcoming.

x   Zambia's parliament had 135 seats in the pre-AIDS era. This was increased to 150 in 1990. Eight extra seats are reserved for nominated candidates, bringing the total to 158 seats.

xi   Malawi has a parliament of 193 seats.

xii   According to the Electoral Commission of Zambia's Deputy Director, Priscilla Isaacs, (telephone interview, 2004).

xiii   Some records show a figure of 6.7 million registered at this time.

xiv   Kapembwa Simbao, (former) Deputy Minister of Health, Zambia, in his opening speech at the IDASA/FODEP/INESOR policy forum on AIDS and elections, 2005.

www.ingramcontent.com/pod-product-compliance
Lightning Source LLC
Chambersburg PA
CBHW080427270326
41929CB00018B/3199